Kale YEAH! Detox and Look Radiant!
20 Easy Juice Recipes with Healing Herbs

By Sherry Inman

ISBN-13: 978-1544920269

ISBN-10: 1544920261

Table of Contents

Introduction

Congratulations on making yourself a priority today! Imagine having more energy and vitality to do all the things you really want to do! Taking time to learn new ways to enhance your diet and take care of yourself is most definitely time well spent. Plus, giving your body more of what it needs to get that wonderfully healthy glow is so worth it. Juicing can help you detox and lose weight while having a significantly positive impact on your vision, skin, and digestive system. Juicing at home is a great way to bring beautiful live fruit, vegetables, and herbs into your everyday life and your body. Just think, it takes about 9 servings to get the recommended daily allowance of fruit and vegetables, which is quite a lot to eat, and juicing makes it easy! Adding juice to your diet may even reduce your risk of illness or serious disease. Supplementing children and growing teens with fresh juice is a great way to deliver extra or missing nutrients from their diet.

Just keep in mind that your juices won't keep very long, so you'll want to drink them within 1-2 days. Each recipe takes about 5 minutes and makes about two 8 oz. servings, depending on the size of your produce. Be sure to include these super nutritious recipes alongside a healthy diet! For suggestions on plant-based meals, check out our food blog and other e-books at freshexpresskitchen.com. We hope you love the recipes in this book and encourage you to come up with some of your own!

~Sherry

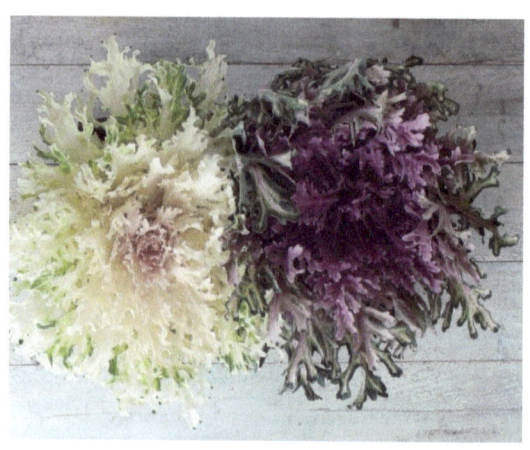

KALE - The nutritional powerhouse of kale is a great detox and super food that is high in iron which is essential for good health, such as cell growth, proper liver function and transporting oxygen to various parts of the body. It is also high in Vitamin K which is necessary for a wide variety of bodily functions including normal bone health and blood clotting. It is an excellent anti-inflammatory food which helps with autoimmune disorders and arthritis and is very high in vitamin A which is great for vision and skin. Surprisingly high in vitamin C, it is very helpful for the metabolism, immune system, and maintaining hydration. It has more calcium than milk, which aids in preventing bone loss, preventing osteoporosis and maintaining a healthy metabolism. It is a great source of omega-fatty acid that is essential for brain health.

Super Foods!

Apples - may improve neurological health, prevent dementia, breast cancer, obesity and its associated disorders and more.

Beets - packed with essential nutrients, beetroots are a great source of fiber, folate, manganese, potassium, iron and vitamin C. Beet juice has been associated with numerous health benefits, including lower blood pressure, improved blood flow and increased exercise performance.

Basil - contains disease-fighting antioxidants, acts as an anti-inflammatory, fights cancer, contains antibacterial properties, contains antimicrobial properties that fight viruses and infections, and promotes cardiovascular health.

Carrots - are a good source of antioxidants, rich in vitamin A, vitamin C, Vitamin K, vitamin B8, pantothenic acid, folate, potassium, iron, copper, and manganese. Carrots have the ability to increase the health of your skin, boost the immune system, improve digestion, increase cardiovascular health, detoxify the body, and boost oral health.

Coconut Water - contains five essential electrolytes that are present in the human body (calcium, magnesium, phosphorous, potassium and sodium). It may lower blood pressure, increase weight loss, increase athletic performance, boost energy, lower cholesterol, reduce cellulite, and relax muscle tension.

Celery - is high in vitamin A, and an excellent source of vitamins B1, B2, B6 and C with rich supplies of potassium, folate, calcium, magnesium, iron, phosphorus, sodium and plenty of essential amino acids. Nutrients in the fiber are released during juicing, aiding in elimination and reducing inflammation. The important minerals in this magical juice effectively balance the body's blood pH, neutralizing acidity.

Cranberries - are a very good source of vitamin C, dietary fiber, and manganese, as well as a good source of vitamin E, vitamin K, copper and pantothenic acid.   The health benefits of cranberry juice may aid in relief from respiratory disorders, urinary tract infection, kidney stones, cancer, and heart disease. It is also beneficial in preventing stomach disorders, diabetes, and gum disease caused by dental plaque.

Ginger - has been used to aid digestion, reduce nausea, help fight the flu and common cold, reduce muscle pain and may drastically lower blood sugar. Reduces oxidative stress and chronic inflammation that can reduce the aging process. Ginger may also be effective against respiratory infections. A little bit goes a long way.

Lemons - are naturally high in Vitamin C, may help to reduce cardiovascular disease, cancer, and the risk of stroke, especially among people who are overweight or have high blood pressure. Lemons aid in digestion and detoxification, they fight damage caused by free radicals, and keep skin looking fresh by producing collagen. I love lemons!

Parsley - high source of antioxidants, it helps protect DNA from damage, can be used as a natural diuretic to help relieve water retention and ease bloating, may help fight kidney stones, UTI and gallbladder infections, improves digestion, benefits skin and dental health by fighting off infections and bacteria, helps to balance hormones that are important for all stages of life including fertility and preventing PMS symptoms.

Spinach - may benefit eye health, reduce oxidative stress, help prevent cancer and reduce blood pressure levels.

Turmeric - is a natural anti-inflammatory compound that helps the body fight foreign invaders, has a role in repairing damage and increases the antioxidant capacity of the body.

Tips for Juicing

1. Buy organic fruits and vegetables if at all possible.
2. Rinse everything well, remove all grocery labels and sticky glue.
3. Discard or remove all imperfections like bruises and brown spots.
4. Have everything precut and ready to go.
5. Roll or fold up your greens and then insert into the feed tube for most juice.
6. Never load the tube when the machine is off. According to manufacturer instructions, it is hard on the motor and will wear down your machine.
7. Follow your juicer instructions and clean your machine well after every use.
8. Store juice in an airtight container to prevent oxidation.
9. For a sweeter juice simply add stevia or your favorite natural sweetener.

Measurements in Recipes

Measurements are approximate as all fruits and vegetables are proportioned differently depending on many factors including crop and location.

1/2 cucumber = 4 oz.

1/2 bunch of celery = 6 oz.

3 medium zucchini = 8 oz.

1 bunch of kale = 3 - 4 oz.

4 medium to large carrots = 4 - 6 oz.

4 small beets = 8 oz. or 1 large beet = 8 oz.

1 head romaine = 4 oz.

1 medium to large apple = 4 - 6 oz.

1 bunch of spinach = 2 oz.

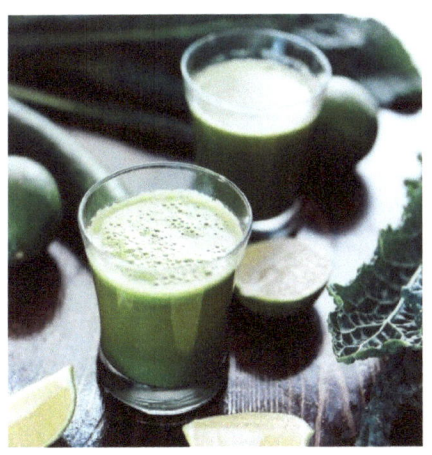

Bazooka Juice

1/2 head romaine lettuce

3 kale leaves

1 cup packed baby spinach

1/2 cucumber

1 zucchini

1/2 cup packed parsley

1 celery stalk

1/2 bunch cilantro

1 large red crispy apple

Juice all ingredients and serve.

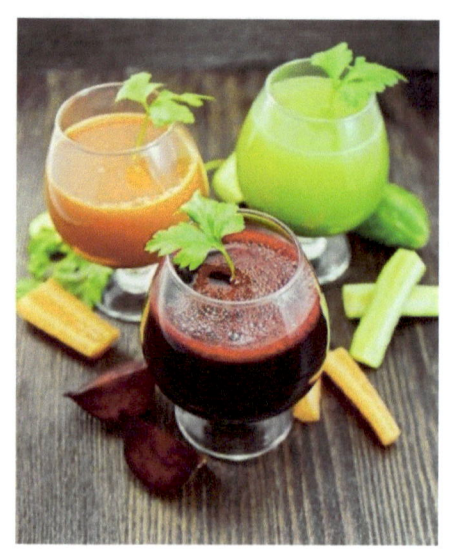

Beet Juice

1 large red apple

1 large beet, leaves & stems

1 large cucumber

2 turmeric roots

Juice all produce, stir and serve.

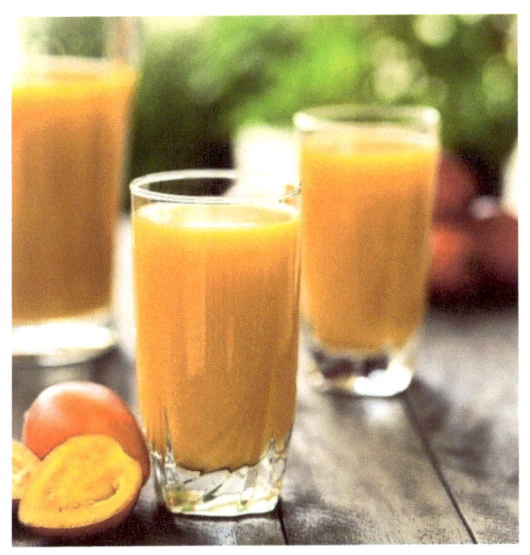

Carrot Juice

7 large carrots

1 large red apple

1 celery stalk

1 cucumber

2" turmeric roots

Juice all produce, stir and serve.

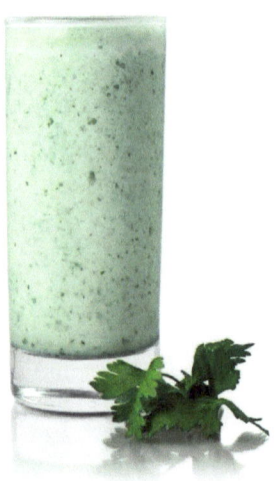

Cilantro Cucumber Juice

1 green apple

2 stalks celery

2 large kale leaves

1 med cucumber

1/4 cup fresh cilantro

1 lemon, peeled

Juice all produce, stir and serve.

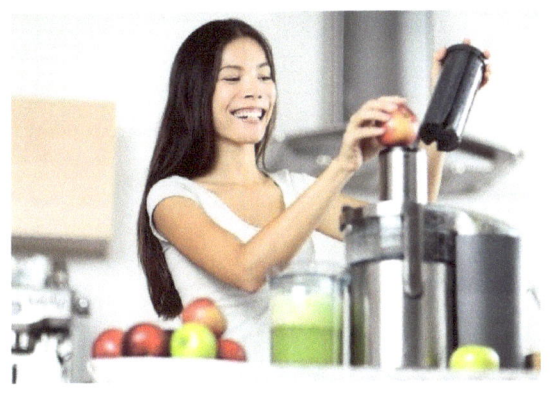

Coconut Limeade

1 cup coconut water

1 large cucumber

1 lime, peeled

1 large red or green apple

Juice all produce, stir and serve.

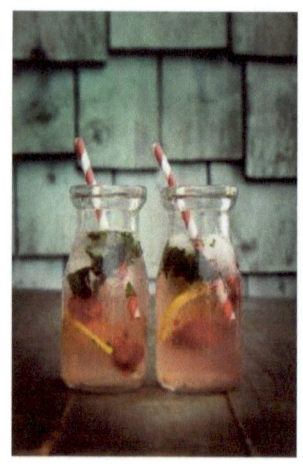

Cranberry Cocktail

1/2 cup cranberries

1 large apple

1 large cucumber

1/2 tablespoon mint leaf

4 whole raspberries

Juice cranberries, apple and cucumber.
Stir in mint, raspberries and serve.

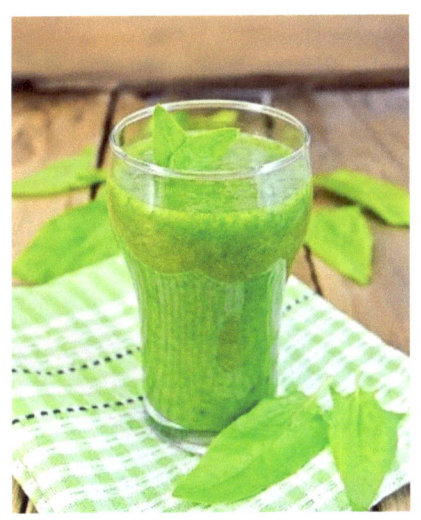

Cucumber Basil Juice

1 cup fresh basil leaves

1 large cucumber

1 lime, peeled

1 green apple

Juice all produce, stir and serve.

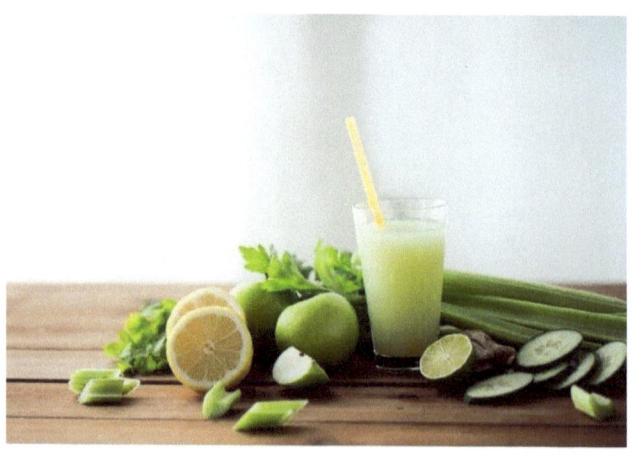

Cucumber Parsley Juice

1 large cucumber

1 med pear

1 green apple

1/2 cup fresh parsley

1 lemon, peeled

2 cups baby spinach

Juice all produce, stir and serve.

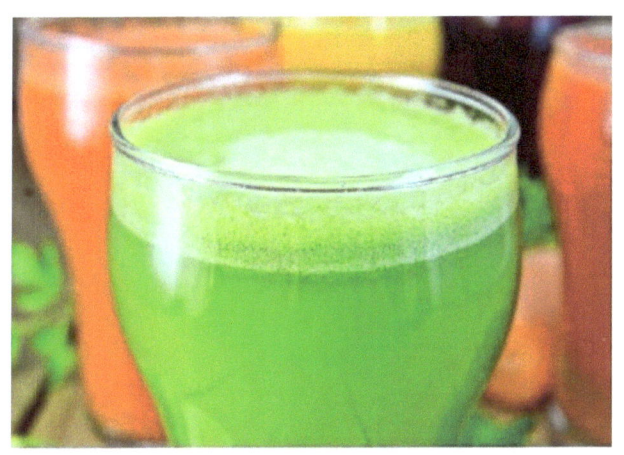

Green Apple Elixir

4 oz. coconut water

3 leaves kale

1 cup spinach, packed

1 large cucumber

1 crisp green apple, cored

2 stalks celery

*Juice all produce. Combine with
coconut water and mix until smooth.*

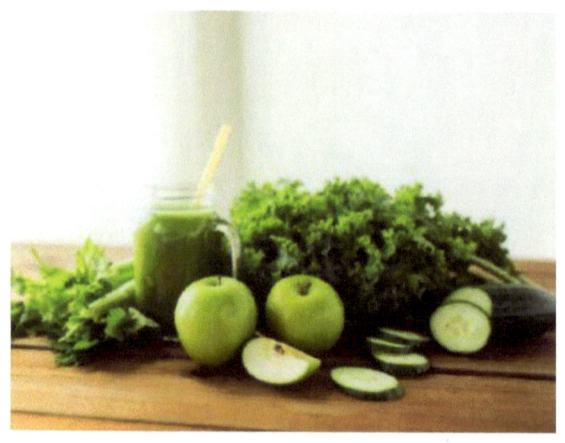

Green Goddess Nectar

3 Stalks of celery

1 bunch of kale

1 large cucumber

1 medium green apple

1 medium pear

Juice all produce, stir and serve.

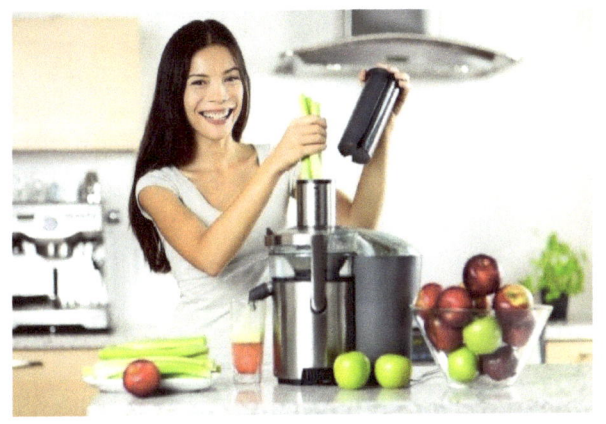

Kale Yeah Detox Juice

1 large green apple

1/2 bunch fresh spinach

2 leaves kale with stalks

1 large cucumber

1 celery stalk

1 lemon

2 oz. coconut water

Juice all produce, add coconut water,
stir and serve.

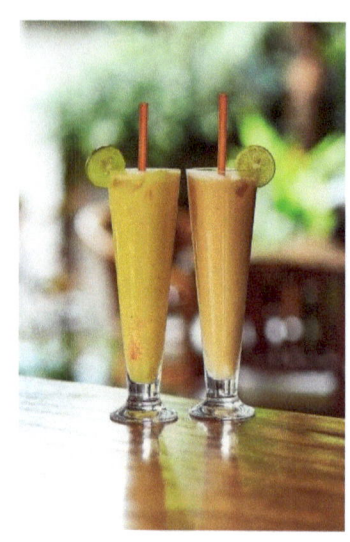

Lemon Zinger

6 large carrots

1 large red apple

1 large lemon

4 oz. coconut water

1/2" of fresh ginger, peeled

1" fresh turmeric

Juice all produce, stir and serve.

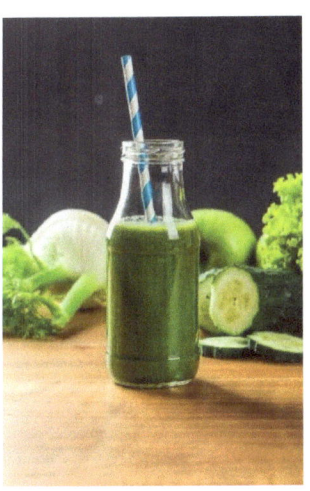

Mean Green Juice

4 oz. coconut water

1 bunch kale leaves & stalks

1 medium cucumber

2" ring large pineapple, cored

1/2 organic lemon with rind

*Juice all produce, stir in coconut water
and serve.*

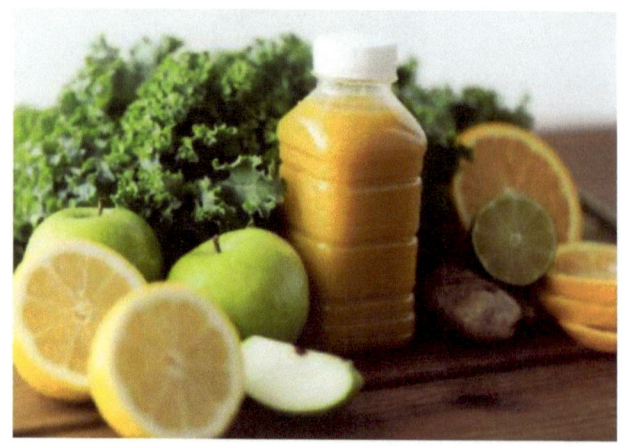

Orange Spinach Juice

2 cups fresh baby spinach

2 large green apples

1 lemon, peeled

2 large oranges, peeled

1 celery stalk

1/2 inch fresh ginger

*Juice all produce, stir
and serve.*

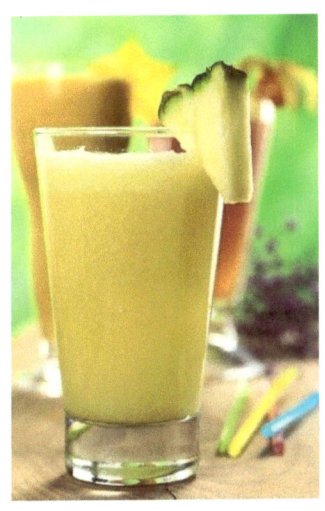

Pineapple Surprise

1 lime, squeezed

1 large cucumber

2 cups pineapple

1 cup coconut water

2 turmeric roots

Juice all produce, add coconut water,

stir and serve.

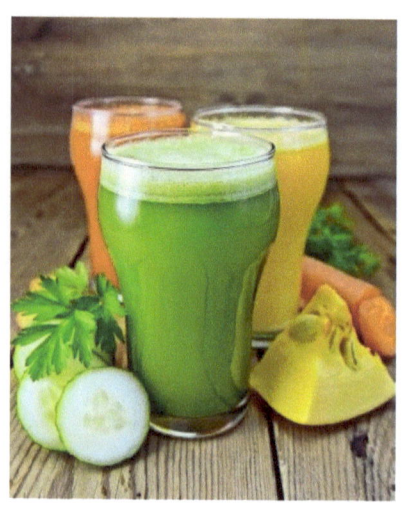

Sunshine Detox Juice

1 rib of celery

1 cup packed cilantro

1 bunch kale leaves with stalks

1 medium cucumber

1" slice pineapple

1/2 large lemon

1" section of fresh ginger, peeled

3 oz. coconut water

Juice all produce, stir & serve.

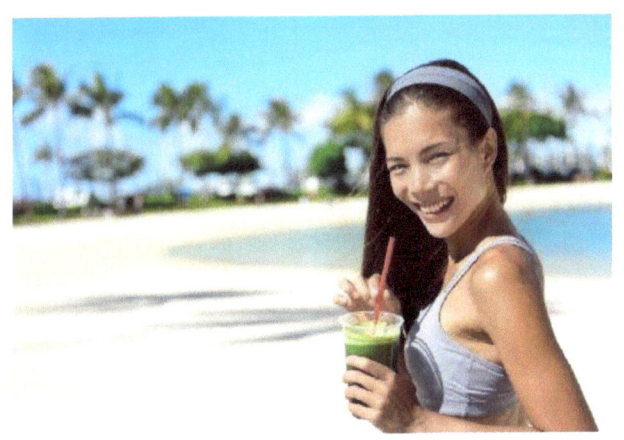

Swiss Chard Lemonade

2 leaves Swiss chard

2 leaves kale

1 med pear

1 large lemon, peeled

1 large cucumber

2 green apples

Juice all produce, stir and serve.

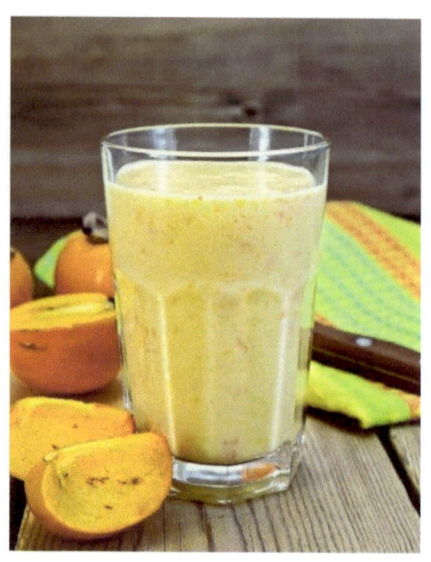

Tampico Slush

6 oz. coconut water

2 oranges, peeled

1 large cucumber

1 lime, peeled

1 cup of crushed ice

*Juice all produce, add coconut water
and ice, mix well and serve.*

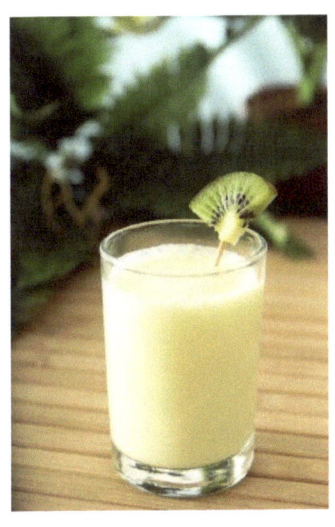

Tropical Escape

2 cups pineapple

2 celery stalks

1 large cucumber

1/2 lemon

1/2 lime

1" piece of fresh ginger

Juice all produce, stir and serve.

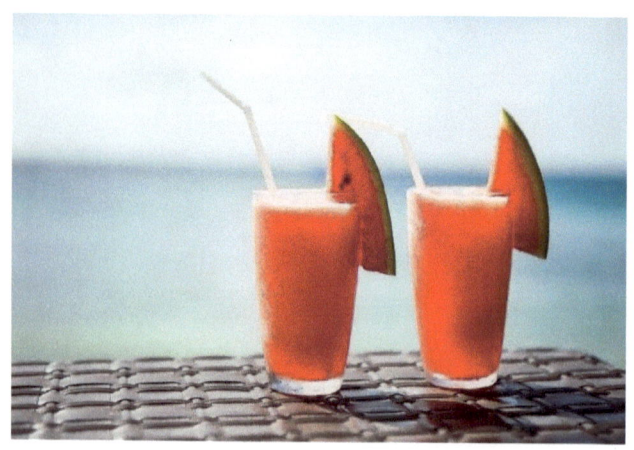

Watermelon Blitz

4 cups cubed seeded watermelon

1/2 cup coconut water

1/2 baby lime

1/2 cucumber

Juice all produce, stir and serve.

Thank you!

Other vegan books:

Easy Vegan Salad Dressings with NutriBullet

By Sherry Inman

Subscribe to our "Amazon Author Page" for new

releases!

www.amazon.com/author/sherryinman

Please visit our online Vegan Recipe Collection!

www.Freshexpresskitchen.com